WONDERS OF ALOE VERA

Complete Guide to Aloe Vera for Health

By

Olagunju oluwagbemiga

TABLE OF CONTENTS

CHAPTER 5

INTRODUCTION

Aloe vera is a succulent plant species that is widely known for its medicinal, cosmetic, and ornamental uses. It belongs to the genus Aloe, and the most commonly cultivated and utilised species is Aloe barbadensis miller. Native to the Arabian Peninsula, Aloe vera has been cultivated and used by various cultures for centuries

Aloe vera's prominence in modern times can be attributed to its manifold applications in both cosmetics and medicine. The plant's gel, extracted from the inner leaf, stands as a testament to nature's pharmacy. Its medicinal applications extend to dermatology, where Aloe vera gel is renowned for its ability to soothe and heal the skin. It is a first-aid remedy for sunburns, minor burns, and skin irritations, providing relief and promoting healing.

In this book you will see how you can use Aloe Vera for your own benefits.

CHAPTER 1

Historical Origin Of Aloe Vera

The historical origin of Aloe vera dates back thousands of years, intertwining with various civilizations, cultures, and regions across the globe. This resilient succulent has been revered for its medicinal, cosmetic, and even spiritual significance, leaving an indelible mark on the tapestry of human history.

The use of Aloe vera can be traced to ancient civilizations, where it held a prominent place in the pharmacopoeias of diverse cultures. In Mesopotamia, one of the cradles of human civilization, clay tablets from around 2100 BCE mention the use of Aloe vera for its healing properties. Similarly, ancient Egyptian papyri dating back to 1550 BCE, including the famous Ebers Papyrus, document the use of Aloe vera for various ailments.

In Egypt, Aloe vera earned the moniker "the plant of immortality" due to its association with life and healing. It was highly prized, and both Cleopatra and Nefertiti were believed to have incorporated Aloe vera into their beauty regimens.

Aloe vera's journey continued eastward, finding its place in ancient Indian and

Chinese medicinal practices. Ayurvedic texts, foundational to traditional Indian medicine, mention the therapeutic uses of Aloe vera for digestive issues, skin disorders, and more. Similarly, traditional Chinese medicine incorporated Aloe vera for its purported healing properties, recognizing its potential to address a range of health concerns.

The knowledge of Aloe vera transcended continents, reaching the ancient Greeks and Romans. The Greek physician Dioscorides, in the 1st century CE, documented the plant's use in his seminal work "De Materia Medica." Aloe vera was utilised as a purgative and skin treatment, highlighting its versatility in addressing both internal and external health concerns.

The Romans, renowned for their adoption and adaptation of diverse cultural practices, embraced Aloe vera for its therapeutic value. It found a place in Roman bathhouses, where individuals would use Aloe vera to soothe and moisturise their skin after bathing.

As the Middle Ages unfolded, the knowledge of Aloe vera persisted. Islamic scholars, during the Golden Age of Islam, played a pivotal role in preserving and advancing medical knowledge. Ibn Sina, also known as Avicenna, an influential

Persian polymath of the 11th century, extolled the virtues of Aloe vera in his medical writings, emphasising its applications in treating wounds and skin conditions.

The Age of Exploration brought Aloe vera to the attention of European explorers and colonists. Spanish and Portuguese explorers encountered the plant in their travels and recognized its potential benefits. The Spanish brought Aloe vera to the Americas, where it found a place in the botanical gardens of the New World.

During the Renaissance, the revival of interest in classical knowledge sparked a renewed fascination with herbal remedies. European botanists and physicians revisited ancient texts, including those mentioning Aloe vera, contributing to its continued popularity.

In the 19th century, as scientific inquiry and botanical studies advanced, Aloe vera drew the attention of botanists and researchers. Aloe vera's introduction to the Western world as a potted plant for homes and gardens further solidified its presence in everyday life.

The early 20th century saw increased scientific interest in Aloe vera's chemical composition and potential applications.

Researchers began to isolate and study the plant's active compounds, contributing to a deeper understanding of its medicinal properties.

In the latter half of the 20th century and into the 21st century, Aloe vera has become a global phenomenon. Its applications have expanded beyond traditional medicine to include cosmetics, skincare, and dietary supplements. The gel extracted from Aloe vera leaves became a popular ingredient in various products, from sunscreens to moisturisers.

Scientific research has sought to validate traditional uses and explore new potential applications. Aloe vera's anti-inflammatory, antioxidant, and wound-healing properties have been subjects of numerous studies, contributing to its continued popularity in modern health and wellness.

Today, Aloe vera is cultivated worldwide, with major producers including countries in Africa, Asia, and the Americas. Its versatility and historical significance have made it a plant of enduring importance, embraced by cultures old and new for its contributions to health, beauty, and well-being. The journey of Aloe vera through the annals of history is a testament to the enduring human fascination with plants and their myriad benefits.

CHAPTER 2

Nutritional Value Of Aloe Vera

Aloe vera is primarily known for its gel, which is used for various medicinal and cosmetic purposes. While it is not commonly consumed as a food, the gel does contain some nutritional components. It's important to note that the nutritional composition can vary based on factors such as:

- The plant's age
- Growing conditions
- A processing methods.

Here are some general aspects of the nutritional value of aloe vera:

1. **Water Content:**
   - Aloe vera gel has a high water content, contributing to its hydrating and moisturising properties.
2. **Vitamins:**
   - Vitamin C: Aloe vera gel may contain small amounts of vitamin C, which is an antioxidant that plays a role in skin health and immune function.
   - Vitamin E: This fat-soluble vitamin with antioxidant properties may also be present in small quantities.
3. **Minerals:**
   - Calcium: Aloe vera gel might contain trace amounts of calcium, which is essential for bone health.

- o Magnesium: Magnesium, involved in various physiological processes, may be present in small amounts.

4. **Enzymes:**
   - o Aloe vera gel contains enzymes such as amylase and lipase, which may aid in the digestion of sugars and fats.

5. **Amino Acids:**
   - o Aloe vera gel contains some amino acids, the building blocks of proteins. While it does not provide complete proteins, the presence of amino acids contributes to its nutritional profile.

6. **Polysaccharides:**
   - o Aloe vera contains complex carbohydrates known as polysaccharides. These compounds are believed to

contribute to the plant's therapeutic properties, including its ability to soothe and moisturize the skin.

7. **Phytochemicals:**
   - Aloe vera contains various phytochemicals, including anthraquinones, which have been studied for their potential therapeutic effects. However, the use of certain anthraquinones, such as aloin, is regulated due to potential side effects.

It's important to highlight that while aloe vera gel may contain some beneficial components, the plant also contains compounds that can be harmful if not used appropriately. The outer leaf skin contains latex, which can have laxative effects and may be associated with adverse reactions. When considering the nutritional value of aloe vera, it's crucial to focus on products specifically designed for consumption and to exercise caution with home-prepared remedies.

As with any supplement or natural remedy, it's advisable to consult with a healthcare professional before incorporating aloe vera products into your diet or skincare routine, especially if you have pre-existing health conditions or are taking medications.

CHAPTER 3

Medicinal Benefits of Aloe Vera:

Aloe vera has been recognized for its medicinal properties for centuries, and its gel, extracted from the inner leaf, is widely used in traditional and modern medicine. While scientific research is ongoing, here are some potential medicinal benefits of aloe vera

1. Skin Health:

    o   *Sunburn Relief:* Aloe vera gel is renowned for its ability to soothe and cool sunburned skin. Its anti-

inflammatory properties can
aid in reducing redness and
discomfort.

- *Wound Healing:* Aloe vera
  may promote the healing of
  minor wounds and burns,
  potentially accelerating the
  skin's recovery process.

2. Moisturization and Hydration:

- *Skincare:* Aloe vera is
  commonly used in cosmetic
  products for its moisturizing
  and hydrating effects. It can
  be beneficial for dry or
  irritated skin.

3. Anti-Inflammatory Effects:

- *Skin Conditions:* Aloe vera may help alleviate symptoms of inflammatory skin conditions, such as eczema and psoriasis, due to its anti-inflammatory properties.

4. Oral Health:

   - *Gum Health:* Some toothpaste and mouthwash formulations include aloe vera for its potential benefits in promoting gum health.

5. Digestive Aid:

   - *Constipation:* Aloe latex, derived from the outer leaf

skin, has been traditionally used as a laxative. However, its use is controversial, and its consumption should be approached with caution due to potential side effects.

6. Antioxidant Properties:

    o *Free Radical Scavenging:* Aloe vera contains antioxidants, such as vitamins C and E, which may help neutralize free radicals in the body.

7. Amino Acids and Enzymes:

    o *Digestion:* Aloe vera contains enzymes that may

aid in the digestion of sugars and fats. It also provides some amino acids, although it is not a significant source of complete proteins.

8. Potential Antimicrobial Effects:

    o *Wound Care:* Aloe vera has been studied for its potential antimicrobial properties, which may contribute to its use in wound care.

    o may help prevent infections when applied to wounds.

9. Inflammatory Bowel Diseases:

    o *Preliminary Studies:* Some studies have explored the

potential use of aloe vera in the management of inflammatory bowel diseases (IBD), such as ulcerative colitis, though more research is needed.

10. Joint and Muscle Pain:

   - *Topical Application:* Aloe vera gel may be applied topically to soothe joint and muscle pain, providing relief from minor discomfort.

11. Skin Conditions:

   - Aloe vera is used to soothe and alleviate symptoms of various skin conditions, including itching and

inflammation.

12. Acne Treatment:

- o Aloe vera gel may be used

  in skincare routines to help

  reduce inflammation and

  promote healing in acne-

  prone skin.

13. Scalp Health:

- o Aloe vera is found in some

  shampoos and conditioners,

  contributing to scalp health

  and promoting healthy hair.

14. Minor Burns and Cuts:

- o Aloe vera gel can be applied

  to minor burns and cuts to

soothe pain and aid in
healing.

15. Immune System Support:

- o Antioxidants in aloe vera
  may contribute to overall
  immune system support.

16. Allergy Relief:

- o Some individuals use aloe
  vera to alleviate skin
  irritations and itching
  associated with allergies.

17. Dental Health:

- o Aloe vera may help in
  maintaining healthy teeth
  and gums when included in
  oral hygiene products.

18. Hemorrhoid Relief:

  o Aloe vera gel applied
    topically may provide relief
    for symptoms associated
    with haemorrhoids.

19. Minor Infections:

  o Due to its potential
    antimicrobial properties,
    aloe vera may be used to aid
    in the healing of minor skin
    infections

20. Sunburn Relief:

  o Aloe vera gel is known for
    its soothing properties,

providing relief to
sunburned skin.

It's important to note that while aloe vera has a long history of traditional use and some promising research findings, more scientific studies are needed to fully understand its mechanisms of action and therapeutic potential. Additionally, the quality and purity of aloe vera products can vary, so it's advisable to use reputable sources and consult with healthcare professionals, especially if considering internal consumption or for individuals with specific health conditions.

Side Effects and Considerations:

1. **Laxative Effect:**

   o *Aloe Latex:* The outer leaf skin contains a substance known as aloe latex, which has strong laxative effects. Prolonged or excessive consumption of aloe latex can lead to dehydration, diarrhea, and electrolyte imbalances.

2. **Allergic Reactions:**

   o *Skin Sensitivity:* Some individuals may be sensitive or allergic to aloe vera, leading to skin irritation or redness. It's advisable to

perform a patch test before
applying aloe vera topically.

3. **Interactions with Medications:**

    o *Drug Interactions:* Aloe
    vera may interact with
    certain medications, such as
    diuretics, anti-diabetes
    drugs, and laxatives.
    Consultation with a
    healthcare professional is
    essential, especially for
    those on medication.

4. **Not Suitable for Internal
Consumption by Everyone:**

    o *Children and Pregnant
    Women:* Aloe latex is not

recommended for children, pregnant women, and individuals with certain medical conditions due to its potential adverse effects.

5. **Quality and Purity Concerns:**

   - ***Commercial Products:*** The quality and purity of aloe vera products can vary. Some commercial products may contain additives or lack the therapeutic properties associated with pure aloe vera gel.

It's crucial to exercise caution and seek professional advice before using aloe vera, particularly for internal consumption or if you have underlying health conditions. While aloe vera has various potential benefits, its improper use can lead to adverse effects. Individual responses may vary, and it's wise to consult with a healthcare provider to ensure safe and effective use based on individual health circumstances.

CHAPTER 4

Aloe Vera Gel and Aloe Vera juice

Aloe Vera Gel:

Aloe vera gel is a thick, clear substance derived from the inner leaf of the Aloe vera plant. It is widely known for its various medicinal and cosmetic uses. The extraction process typically involves filleting the inner part of the leaf to obtain the gel. Aloe vera gel has a gelatinous texture, is usually clear or slightly yellowish, and has a mild, fresh scent. Aloe vera gel is also a common ingredient in cosmetic products like lotions, creams, and sunscreens.

Aloe Vera Juice:

Aloe vera juice is a liquid extract made from the gel of the Aloe vera plant. The juice is obtained by crushing or grinding the inner fillet of the Aloe vera leaf. It is typically clear or slightly yellowish and has a liquid consistency. Aloe vera juice is distinct from the gel in that it is a liquid form, making it suitable for internal consumption. It is consumed for various reasons, including potential digestive benefits, hydration, and as a source of certain vitamins and minerals.

Some aloe vera juices may include sweeteners or flavourings to improve taste, and they are available in various formulations on the market.

Key Points:

- Application: Aloe vera gel is primarily used topically for skincare, while aloe vera juice is suitable for internal consumption.
- Texture: Gel is thicker and more gelatinous, while juice has a liquid consistency.
- Use Cases: Aloe vera gel is commonly used for sunburn relief, wound healing, and skincare,

while aloe vera juice may be consumed for potential digestive benefits and hydration.

Tips For Consuming Aloe Vera Juice

Consuming aloe vera juice can offer potential health benefits, but it's essential to do so in a mindful and cautious manner.

Here are some tips for safely incorporating aloe vera juice into your routine:

1. **Choose High-Quality Products:**
   - Opt for aloe vera juice from reputable brands or sources

that prioritise quality and purity. Read product labels to ensure that it's specifically intended for internal consumption.

2. **Check for Additives:**

    o   Be mindful of additional ingredients, such as sweeteners or flavourings, especially if you have dietary restrictions or preferences. Choose products with minimal additives.

3. **Start with Small Amounts:**

- Begin with a small amount, especially if you are new to consuming aloe vera juice. This allows you to assess your body's response and potential tolerance.

4. **Consult with Healthcare Professionals:**

   - Before incorporating aloe vera juice into your routine, consult with your healthcare provider, especially if you have pre-existing health conditions, are pregnant, or are taking medications. They can provide

personalised advice based
on your health status.

5. **Avoid Aloe Latex:**

   o Aloe latex, found in the
   outer leaf skin, has strong
   laxative effects and may
   cause adverse reactions.
   Choose aloe vera juice
   products that are processed
   to remove or minimise aloe
   latex content.

6. **Monitor for Allergic Reactions:**

   o Perform a patch test before
   consuming larger amounts
   to check for any potential
   allergic reactions. This is

particularly important if you have known allergies to plants or other substances.

7. **Limit Consumption:**

   o Consume aloe vera juice in moderation. While it may offer potential health benefits, excessive consumption may lead to adverse effects, including diarrhoea or dehydration.

8. **Time of Consumption:**

   o Some people prefer to consume aloe vera juice on an empty stomach in the morning. However, individual preferences and tolerances vary, so find a time that works best for you.

9. **Stay Hydrated:**

   - Aloe vera juice can contribute to your overall fluid intake. However, it's essential to maintain proper hydration by drinking an adequate amount of water throughout the day.

10. **Observe Individual Tolerance:**

    - Pay attention to how your body responds to aloe vera juice. If you experience any discomfort, digestive issues,

or allergic reactions,
discontinue use and consult
with a healthcare
professional.

11. **Combine with Other**
    Ingredients:

    - If the taste of aloe vera juice
      is not to your liking,
      consider blending it with
      other ingredients, such as
      fruit juices or smoothies, to
      enhance flavour.

Remember that individual responses to aloe vera juice can vary, and what works for one person may not work for another. It's crucial to prioritise your health and well-being by making informed choices and seeking professional advice when needed.

Tips for using aloe vera gel

Aloe vera gel is a versatile substance with various applications for skincare and minor health concerns. Here are some tips for using aloe vera gel effectively and safely:

1. **Choose Pure Aloe Vera Gel:**
   - Opt for high-quality, pure aloe vera gel with minimal additives. Check the ingredient list to ensure it does not contain unnecessary fillers, colourants, or fragrances.

2. **Perform a Patch Test:**

    - Before applying aloe vera
      gel to a larger area of your
      skin, perform a patch test on
      a small, inconspicuous area
      to check for any allergic
      reactions or sensitivities.

3. **Sunburn Relief:**

    - Aloe vera gel is renowned
      for its soothing properties.
      Apply it to sunburned areas
      for relief from pain and
      inflammation. Keep the gel
      in the refrigerator for an
      additional cooling effect.

4. **Wound Healing:**

o   Use aloe vera gel on minor cuts, wounds, or burns to promote healing. Clean the affected area first, then apply a thin layer of the gel.

5. **Skin Moisturiser:**

   o   Apply aloe vera gel as a natural moisturiser for your face and body. It hydrates the skin without clogging pores, making it suitable for various skin types.

6. **Acne Treatment:**

   o   Aloe vera gel can be used on acne-prone skin to reduce inflammation and redness. It may also aid in healing acne scars.

7. **Hair and Scalp Treatment:**

   - Massage aloe vera gel into your scalp to soothe irritation and promote a healthy scalp. You can also apply it to your hair as a conditioner to add moisture and reduce frizz.

8. **After Shaving:**

   - Use aloe vera gel as an aftershave to soothe irritation and prevent razor burns. Its cooling properties

can provide relief to
sensitive skin.

9. **Eye Makeup Remover:**

    o Apply a small amount of
       aloe vera gel to a cotton pad
       and use it to gently remove
       eye makeup. It is gentle and
       hydrating for the delicate
       skin around the eyes.

10. **Anti-Itch Treatment:**

    o Apply aloe vera gel to insect
       bites, rashes, or itchy skin
       for relief. Its anti-
       inflammatory properties can
       help alleviate itching.

11. **DIY Face Masks:**

- Mix aloe vera gel with other
  natural ingredients like
  honey, yoghourt, or clay to
  create homemade face
  masks tailored to your skin's
  needs.

12. **Store Properly:**

- Store your aloe vera gel in a
  cool, dark place, and check
  the expiration date.
  Exposure to heat and light
  can degrade its beneficial
  properties.

13. **Consult with Professionals:**

  - If you have specific skin
    concerns or conditions,
    consult with dermatologists
    or healthcare professionals
    before incorporating aloe
    vera gel into your skincare
    routine.

14. **Hydrate from the Inside:**

  - In addition to topical use,
    staying hydrated and
    maintaining a healthy diet
    contributes to overall skin
    health.

Remember that individual responses to aloe
vera gel can vary, and it's essential to

monitor your skin's reaction. If you experience any adverse effects, discontinue use and consult with a healthcare professional.

CHAPTER 5

Growing and care for your Aloe Vera plant indoors and outdoors

Growing and caring for Aloe vera plants can be rewarding, as they are relatively low-maintenance and have several practical uses. Here are guidelines for cultivating and caring for Aloe vera plants both indoors and outdoors:

Indoor Aloe Vera Care:

1. Potting Mix:

- Use a well-draining potting mix
  specifically designed for
  succulents or cacti. Aloe vera roots
  are prone to rot in soggy soil.

2. Container:

- Choose a pot with drainage holes
  to prevent waterlogging.
  Terracotta or clay pots are good
  choices as they allow excess
  moisture to evaporate.

3. Light:

- Place the Aloe vera near a bright,
  sunny window where it can receive
  indirect sunlight. They prefer

bright light but can tolerate some shade.

4. Watering:

- Allow the soil to dry out between waterings. Overwatering is a common issue; water sparingly, and ensure excess water drains away.

5. Temperature:

- Aloe vera prefers temperatures between 59°F to 77°F (15°C to 25°C). It can tolerate occasional cooler temperatures but should be protected from frost.

6. Fertilisation:

- Fertilise sparingly, usually once every 4-6 weeks during the growing season (spring and summer) with a balanced, diluted fertiliser.

7. Repotting:

- Repot the Aloe vera if it outgrows its container or if the soil becomes depleted. Repotting is typically done every 2-3 years.

8. Pruning:

- Remove any dead or withered leaves at the base using clean, sharp scissors or pruning shears.

Outdoor Aloe Vera Care:

1. Planting Location:

- Choose a well-draining location in the garden with sandy or rocky soil. Ensure good drainage to prevent waterlogging.

2. Sunlight:

- Aloe vera thrives in full sunlight but can tolerate partial shade. Provide at least 6 hours of sunlight per day.

3. Watering:

- Water sparingly, especially during the growing season. Aloe vera is drought-tolerant and prefers slightly dry conditions.

4. Cold Protection:

- If you live in a region with frost, protect the Aloe vera during cold spells by covering it or moving it indoors.

5. Propagation:

- Aloe vera can be propagated by removing offsets (pups) that grow at the base of the plant. Allow the

offset to dry for a day before
planting it in well-draining soil.

6. Pests and Diseases:

- Aloe vera is generally resistant to
  pests and diseases. However,
  overwatering can lead to root rot.
  Watch for signs of pests like
  mealybugs and scale, and treat
  them promptly.

7. Harvesting Aloe Gel:

- If you want to harvest Aloe vera
  gel, select mature leaves, and cut
  them close to the base. Squeeze or
  scrape out the gel for various uses.

8. Pruning:

- Prune dead or damaged leaves with clean, sharp tools to maintain the plant's appearance and health.

General Tips:

- Aloe vera is forgiving of occasional neglect but thrives with consistent care.

- Be cautious with overwatering, as Aloe vera is more tolerant of drought than excess moisture.

- Avoid leaving Aloe vera in standing water, as it can lead to root rot.

By following these guidelines, you can successfully grow and care for Aloe vera plants, whether indoors or outdoors. Adjust care practices based on your specific climate and environmental conditions.

www.ingramcontent.com/pod-product-compliance
Lightning Source LLC
Chambersburg PA
CBHW071105260726
48661CB00006B/2468